NAVIGATING CANCER

A Workbook for Managing Your Cancer Care

DR. THOMAS GRUBER • MARCIA GRUBER-PAGE RN

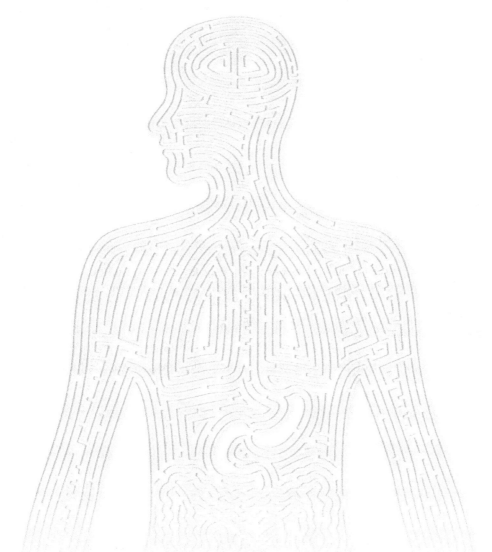

NAVIGATING CANCER

A Workbook for Managing Your Cancer Care

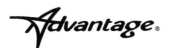

Published by Advantage, Charleston, South Carolina.
Member of Advantage Media Group.

ADVANTAGE is a registered trademark, and the Advantage colophon is a trademark of Advantage Media Group, Inc.

Printed in the United States of America.

10 9 8 7 6 5 4 3 2 1

ISBN: 978-1-64225-911-7 (Paperback)

Designed by Wesley Strickland.

This publication is designed to provide accurate and authoritative information in regard to the subject matter covered. It is sold with the understanding that the publisher is not engaged in rendering legal, accounting, or other professional services. If legal advice or other expert assistance is required, the services of a competent professional person should be sought.

Advantage Media Group is a publisher of business, self-improvement, and professional development books and online learning. We help entrepreneurs, business leaders, and professionals share their Stories, Passion, and Knowledge to help others Learn & Grow. Do you have a manuscript or book idea that you would like us to consider for publishing? Please visit **advantagefamily.com**.

INTRODUCTION

· ·

When I walked past the exam room, I heard a sigh and a tearful sob. I entered the room and asked, "Can I help?" The patient sobbed, "It's too much. I'm scared. What if I forget something? Will I die?" Her husband asked, "How will we ever keep track of all of these appointments and all of her medications? I'm afraid of making a mistake; this is too important."

A gentleman knocked on my office door and asked if I had a three-hole punch that he could borrow. As I walked him over to the clerical station I asked what he needed it for. He pulled a three-ring binder out of his valise and said, "I'm keeping track of my son's test results, appointments, and disability papers for him," and he proudly showed me how he had created the index tabs so that he or his son could find the right sections.

I walked into the clinic reception area, and there was a woman on the floor picking up a stack of papers that she had dropped. I bent down to help her and realized these papers were copies of pathology reports, imaging reports, chemo schedules, a "cancer" diet article from the internet, insurance information, and various other information related to a patient's medical situation. She explained that the patient was her mother who was in the exam room with the doctor. She had dropped all the paperwork when she stood to accompany her mother into the exam room. I told her to go be with her mother and I would bring her all her papers. She asked if I could find a "big rubber band" so that she would not drop the papers again.

"You have cancer." These are the three most terrifying words in any language. They cause a tumult of emotions that range from fear and panic to denial and "why me?" to anger, anxiety, and depression. For most patients, they are so stunned by those words that their ability to hear and understand anything the doctor says after that is limited.

"Now what?" Several actions may be recommended by your doctor when you are first diagnosed and throughout treatment. Your doctor may recommend more diagnostic testing. Your doctor may talk with you about treatment options. Your doctor may refer you to a specialist or two or three.

"How do I remember all of this?" Cancer is a complicated disease, and so are the diagnostic and treatment processes. We have watched our patients and their families struggle to remember and keep track of the multiple appointments, procedures, specialists, test results, co-pays, sick leave, disability applications, and everything else that you take care of for your family and others who depend on you. As described in the real-life examples at the beginning of this introduction, we have seen patients and their families devise many ways to keep track of all the information—stacks of loose papers held together with rubber bands and clips, three-ring binders, black/white composition notebooks, two-ring binders with pockets, plastic supermarket bags, manilla folders, and various combinations of methods as an attempt by our patients and family to keep all their health-related information and reminders in order.

A diagnosis of any type of cancer is frightening, and the journey through diagnosis and treatment is complex and often confusing. *Navigating Cancer: A Workbook for Managing Your Cancer Care,* will walk you through the experience so that you know what to expect. This workbook will help you track, manage, understand, and communicate the information that is important for you to progress through your medical care. The pages in the guide provide an easy way for you to list and organize your doctor and test appointments, treatment schedules, and dates of surgery and procedures. There is also a list of possible side effects for you to track and date, if they occur. "Notes" pages are included, and you can use these for anything you want—questions for the doctor or your innermost thoughts about your experience.

Another side effect of learning that you have cancer is the feeling that your life is spinning out of control and that the cancer is in charge. We created this guide to give you back some of that control.

This workbook is dedicated to my very first Nurse Manager, Mrs. Christine Robinson. Mrs. Robinson told me very early in my career that professional inspiration will come from our patients. She was right! A Workbook for Managing Your Cancer Care *is dedicated to the countless number of courageous patients and their loved ones whom we have cared for during our respective careers. We have observed our patients struggle as they attempt to keep track of the copious amount of information related to their care and their diagnoses. It became clear to us that being able to organize and track their medical care is an important piece of regaining some control for our patients—and for the friends and family who are alongside the patient on this path. We designed this Guide to relieve some of the anxiety and give you back some control.*

PATIENT DEMOGRAPHICS AND MY TEAM

THIS BOOK BELONGS TO:

_____

_____

PHONE #: _____

IN CASE OF EMERGENCY:

_____

_____

PHONE #: _____

PRIMARY CARE DOCTOR:

_____

_____

PHONE #: _____

GYNECOLOGIST/GYNECOLOGIC ONCOLOGIST:

_____

_____

PHONE #: _____

SURGEON:

_____

_____

PHONE #: _____

MEDICAL ONCOLOGIST:

_____

_____

PHONE #: _____

RADIATION ONCOLOGIST:

_____

_____

PHONE #:

_____

UROLOGIST/UROLOGIC ONCOLOGIST:

_____

_____

PHONE #:

_____

PALLIATIVE CARE DOCTOR:

_____

_____

PHONE #:

_____

NURSE NAVIGATOR:

_____

_____

PHONE #:

_____

NURSE PRACTITIONER/PA:

_____

_____

PHONE #:

_____

NURSE PRACTITIONER/PA:

_____

_____

PHONE #:

_____

NURSE PRACTITIONER/PA:

_____

_____

PHONE #: _____

NURSE PRACTITIONER/PA:

_____

_____

PHONE #: _____

OTHER DOCTOR(S):

_____

_____

PHONE #: _____

OTHER DOCTOR(S):

_____

_____

PHONE #: _____

OTHER DOCTOR(S):

_____

_____

PHONE #: _____

ALLERGIES:

_____

_____

_____

NOTES

NOTES

INSURANCE AND PRESCRIPTION DRUG INFORMATION

PRIMARY INSURANCE PROVIDER:

NAME OF POLICY HOLDER:

DOB OF PRIMARY POLICY HOLDER:

MEMBER ID #:   GROUP #:

PLAN TYPE: BENEFITS #:

SECONDARY INSURANCE PROVIDER:

NAME OF POLICY HOLDER:

DOB OF PRIMARY POLICY HOLDER:

MEMBER ID #:   GROUP #:

PLAN TYPE: BENEFITS #:

PRESCRIPTION DRUG ID CARD

PREFERRED PHARMACY:

ADDRESS:

ID #:

RxGRP:

RxBIN:

RxPCN:

PRESCRIPTION DRUG ID CARD

PREFERRED PHARMACY:

ADDRESS:

ID #:

RxGRP:

RxBIN:

RxPCN:

DIAGNOSES INFORMATION:

DIAGNOSES:

DATE OF DIAGNOSIS:

WAS A BIOPSY DONE? ☐ YES ☐ NO   IF YES:

DATE:

WHERE:

RESULTS:

ASK YOUR DOCTOR IF THEY ORDERED ANY GENETIC, GENOMIC, MOLECULAR OR BIOMARKER TESTING? ☐ YES ☐ NO

IF YES, WHAT WAS THE RESULT?:

PRESCRIPTION MEDICATIONS:

DRUG NAME: DOSE:

HOW OFTEN?

REASON:

DOCTOR WHO PRESCRIBED:

DRUG NAME: DOSE:

HOW OFTEN?

REASON:

DOCTOR WHO PRESCRIBED:

DRUG NAME: DOSE:

HOW OFTEN?

REASON:

DOCTOR WHO PRESCRIBED:

DRUG NAME: DOSE:

HOW OFTEN?

REASON:

DOCTOR WHO PRESCRIBED:

PRESCRIPTION MEDICATIONS:

DRUG NAME: _____   DOSE: _____

HOW OFTEN? _____

REASON: _____

DOCTOR WHO PRESCRIBED: _____

DRUG NAME: _____   DOSE: _____

HOW OFTEN? _____

REASON: _____

DOCTOR WHO PRESCRIBED: _____

DRUG NAME: _____   DOSE: _____

HOW OFTEN? _____

REASON: _____

DOCTOR WHO PRESCRIBED: _____

DRUG NAME: _____   DOSE: _____

HOW OFTEN? _____

REASON: _____

DOCTOR WHO PRESCRIBED: _____

PRESCRIPTION MEDICATIONS:

DRUG NAME: _____ DOSE: _____

HOW OFTEN? _____

REASON: _____

DOCTOR WHO PRESCRIBED: _____

DRUG NAME: _____ DOSE: _____

HOW OFTEN? _____

REASON: _____

DOCTOR WHO PRESCRIBED: _____

DRUG NAME: _____ DOSE: _____

HOW OFTEN? _____

REASON: _____

DOCTOR WHO PRESCRIBED: _____

DRUG NAME: _____ DOSE: _____

HOW OFTEN? _____

REASON: _____

DOCTOR WHO PRESCRIBED: _____

PRESCRIPTION MEDICATIONS:

DRUG NAME: _____ DOSE: _____

HOW OFTEN? _____

REASON: _____

DOCTOR WHO PRESCRIBED: _____

DRUG NAME: _____ DOSE: _____

HOW OFTEN? _____

REASON: _____

DOCTOR WHO PRESCRIBED: _____

DRUG NAME: _____ DOSE: _____

HOW OFTEN? _____

REASON: _____

DOCTOR WHO PRESCRIBED: _____

DRUG NAME: _____ DOSE: _____

HOW OFTEN? _____

REASON: _____

DOCTOR WHO PRESCRIBED: _____

OVER-THE-COUNTER MEDICATIONS, VITAMINS, AND HERBAL SUBSTANCES:

DRUG NAME: _____ DOSE: _____

HOW OFTEN? _____

REASON: _____

DRUG NAME: _____ DOSE: _____

HOW OFTEN? _____

REASON: _____

DRUG NAME: _____ DOSE: _____

HOW OFTEN? _____

REASON: _____

DRUG NAME: _____ DOSE: _____

HOW OFTEN? _____

REASON: _____

DRUG NAME: _____ DOSE: _____

HOW OFTEN? _____

REASON: _____

OVER-THE-COUNTER MEDICATIONS, VITAMINS, AND HERBAL SUBSTANCES:

DRUG NAME: _____ DOSE: _____

HOW OFTEN? _____

REASON: _____

DRUG NAME: _____ DOSE: _____

HOW OFTEN? _____

REASON: _____

DRUG NAME: _____ DOSE: _____

HOW OFTEN? _____

REASON: _____

DRUG NAME: _____ DOSE: _____

HOW OFTEN? _____

REASON: _____

DRUG NAME: _____ DOSE: _____

HOW OFTEN? _____

REASON: _____

NOTES

NOTES

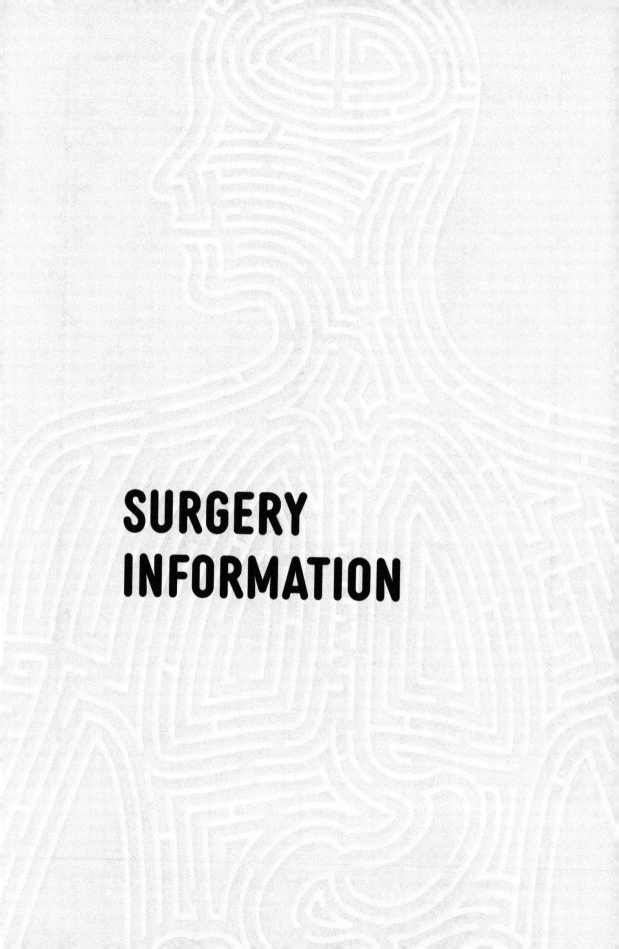

SURGERY INFORMATION

MY SURGERY TEAM

NAME OF SURGERY PRACTICE:
_____

_____

ADDRESS: _____ PHONE: _____

_____

SURGEON: _____ PHONE: _____

_____

NURSE PRACTITIONER: _____ PHONE: _____

_____

PHYSICIAN ASSISTANT: _____ PHONE: _____

_____

NURSE/NURSE NAVIGATOR: _____ PHONE: _____

_____

SCHEDULER: _____ PHONE: _____

_____

PATIENT PORTAL WEBSITE ADDRESS:
_____

_____

ADDITIONAL INFO: _____

_____

SURGERY VISIT SUMMARY

DATE: _____

DOCTOR/PRACTITIONER SEEN: _____

REASON FOR APPOINTMENT: _____

☐ PRE SURGERY EVALUATION   ☐ POST SURGERY FOLLOW UP

☐ OTHER: _____

TESTING DONE FOR THIS APPOINTMENT:
_____
_____

QUESTIONS FOR THE DOCTOR/PRACTITIONER:
_____
_____
_____
_____
_____

SUMMARY OF VISIT

RESULTS OF TESTING:
_____
_____

TESTING ORDERED FOR NEXT VISIT:
_____
_____

MEDICATION CHANGES:
_____
_____

REFERRALS:
_____

SURGERY VISIT SUMMARY

DATE: _____

DOCTOR/PRACTITIONER SEEN: _____

REASON FOR APPOINTMENT: _____

☐ PRE SURGERY EVALUATION   ☐ POST SURGERY FOLLOW UP

☐ OTHER: _____

TESTING DONE FOR THIS APPOINTMENT: _____
_____

QUESTIONS FOR THE DOCTOR/PRACTITIONER: _____
_____
_____
_____
_____

SUMMARY OF VISIT

RESULTS OF TESTING: _____
_____

TESTING ORDERED FOR NEXT VISIT: _____
_____

MEDICATION CHANGES: _____
_____

REFERRALS: _____

SURGERY VISIT SUMMARY

DATE: _____

DOCTOR/PRACTITIONER SEEN: _____

REASON FOR APPOINTMENT: _____

☐ PRE SURGERY EVALUATION   ☐ POST SURGERY FOLLOW UP

☐ OTHER: _____

TESTING DONE FOR THIS APPOINTMENT:

_____

_____

QUESTIONS FOR THE DOCTOR/PRACTITIONER:

_____

_____

_____

_____

SUMMARY OF VISIT

RESULTS OF TESTING:

_____

_____

TESTING ORDERED FOR NEXT VISIT:

_____

_____

MEDICATION CHANGES:

_____

_____

REFERRALS:

_____

SURGERY VISIT SUMMARY

DATE: _____

DOCTOR/PRACTITIONER SEEN: _____

REASON FOR APPOINTMENT: _____

☐ PRE SURGERY EVALUATION   ☐ POST SURGERY FOLLOW UP

☐ OTHER: _____

TESTING DONE FOR THIS APPOINTMENT: _____

_____

QUESTIONS FOR THE DOCTOR/PRACTITIONER: _____

_____

_____

_____

SUMMARY OF VISIT

RESULTS OF TESTING: _____

_____

TESTING ORDERED FOR NEXT VISIT: _____

_____

MEDICATION CHANGES: _____

_____

REFERRALS: _____

SURGERY VISIT SUMMARY

DATE: _____

DOCTOR/PRACTITIONER SEEN: _____

REASON FOR APPOINTMENT: _____

☐ PRE SURGERY EVALUATION   ☐ POST SURGERY FOLLOW UP

☐ OTHER: _____

TESTING DONE FOR THIS APPOINTMENT: _____

_____

QUESTIONS FOR THE DOCTOR/PRACTITIONER: _____

_____

_____

_____

_____

SUMMARY OF VISIT

RESULTS OF TESTING: _____

_____

TESTING ORDERED FOR NEXT VISIT: _____

_____

MEDICATION CHANGES: _____

_____

REFERRALS: _____

SURGERIES AND OTHER PROCEDURES

During the course of your treatment you may have one or more surgeries or procedures to diagnose, treat, assess response to treatment or to manage symptoms. This section has space for you to keep track of those procedures.

DATE: _____

LOCATION: _____

DOCTOR NAME: _____

PROCEDURE: _____

NOTES: _____

_____

_____

DATE: _____

LOCATION: _____

DOCTOR NAME: _____

PROCEDURE: _____

NOTES: _____

_____

_____

SURGERIES AND OTHER PROCEDURES

DATE:
_____

LOCATION:
_____

DOCTOR NAME:
_____

PROCEDURE:
_____

NOTES:
_____

_____

_____

_____

_____

DATE:
_____

LOCATION:
_____

DOCTOR NAME:
_____

PROCEDURE:
_____

NOTES:
_____

_____

_____

_____

SURGERIES AND OTHER PROCEDURES

DATE:
_____

LOCATION:
_____

DOCTOR NAME:
_____

PROCEDURE:
_____

NOTES:
_____

_____

_____

_____

_____

DATE:
_____

LOCATION:
_____

DOCTOR NAME:
_____

PROCEDURE:
_____

NOTES:
_____

_____

_____

_____

SURGERIES AND OTHER PROCEDURES

DATE:
_____

LOCATION:
_____

DOCTOR NAME:
_____

PROCEDURE:
_____

NOTES:
_____

_____

_____

_____

_____

DATE:
_____

LOCATION:
_____

DOCTOR NAME:
_____

PROCEDURE:
_____

NOTES:
_____

_____

_____

_____

SURGERIES AND OTHER PROCEDURES

DATE:
_____

LOCATION:
_____

DOCTOR NAME:
_____

PROCEDURE:
_____

NOTES:
_____

_____

_____

_____

_____

DATE:
_____

LOCATION:
_____

DOCTOR NAME:
_____

PROCEDURE:
_____

NOTES:
_____

_____

_____

_____

SURGERIES AND OTHER PROCEDURES

DATE:
_____

LOCATION:
_____

DOCTOR NAME:
_____

PROCEDURE:
_____

NOTES:
_____

_____

_____

_____

_____

DATE:
_____

LOCATION:
_____

DOCTOR NAME:
_____

PROCEDURE:
_____

NOTES:
_____

_____

_____

_____

NOTES

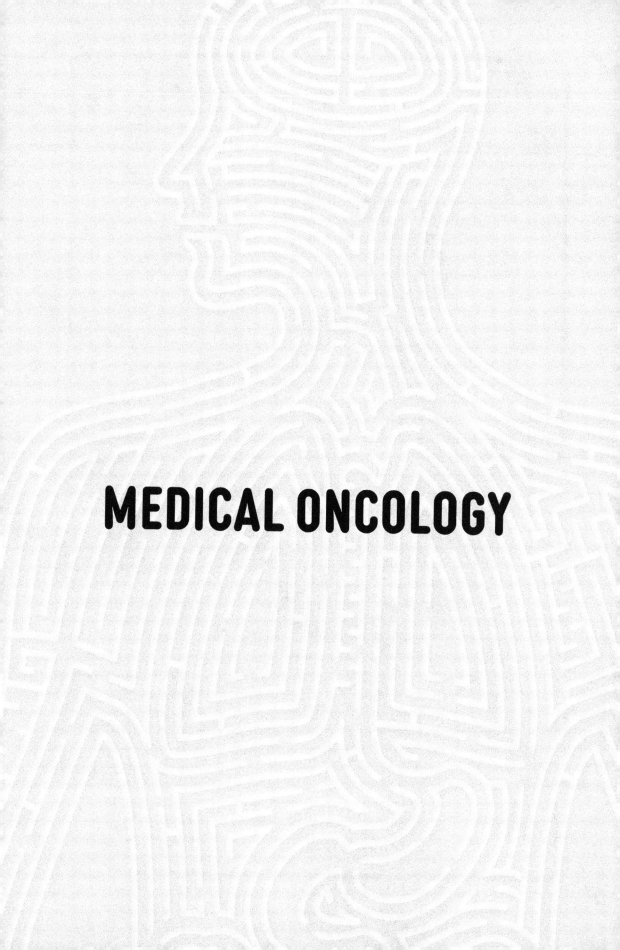

MEDICAL ONCOLOGY

MY MEDICAL ONCOLOGY TEAM

NAME OF ONCOLOGY PRACTICE:

_____

_____

ADDRESS: PHONE:

_____

_____

DOCTOR: PHONE:

_____

_____

NURSE PRACTITIONER: PHONE:

_____

_____

PHYSICIAN ASSISTANT: PHONE:

_____

_____

NURSE/NURSE NAVIGATOR: PHONE:

_____

_____

SCHEDULER: PHONE:

_____

_____

PATIENT PORTAL WEBSITE ADDRESS:

_____

_____

ADDITIONAL INFO:

_____

_____

MEDICAL ONCOLOGY VISIT SUMMARY DATE: _____

DOCTOR/PRACTITIONER SEEN:
_____

REASON FOR APPOINTMENT:
_____

☐ NEW PATIENT VISIT   ☐ ROUTINE FOLLOWUP

☐ URGENT CARE VISIT   ☐ OTHER: _____

TESTING DONE FOR THIS APPOINTMENT:
_____
_____

QUESTIONS FOR THE DOCTOR/PRACTITIONER:
_____
_____
_____
_____

SUMMARY OF VISIT

RESULTS OF TESTING:
_____
_____

TESTING ORDERED FOR NEXT VISIT:
_____
_____

MEDICATION CHANGES:
_____
_____

REFERRALS:
_____

MEDICAL ONCOLOGY VISIT SUMMARY DATE: _____

DOCTOR/PRACTITIONER SEEN: _____

REASON FOR APPOINTMENT: _____

☐ NEW PATIENT VISIT   ☐ ROUTINE FOLLOWUP

☐ URGENT CARE VISIT   ☐ OTHER: _____

TESTING DONE FOR THIS APPOINTMENT: _____

_____

QUESTIONS FOR THE DOCTOR/PRACTITIONER: _____

_____

_____

_____

_____

SUMMARY OF VISIT

RESULTS OF TESTING: _____

_____

TESTING ORDERED FOR NEXT VISIT: _____

_____

MEDICATION CHANGES: _____

_____

REFERRALS: _____

MEDICAL ONCOLOGY VISIT SUMMARY DATE: _____

DOCTOR/PRACTITIONER SEEN: _____

REASON FOR APPOINTMENT: _____

☐ NEW PATIENT VISIT   ☐ ROUTINE FOLLOWUP

☐ URGENT CARE VISIT   ☐ OTHER: _____

TESTING DONE FOR THIS APPOINTMENT:

_____

_____

QUESTIONS FOR THE DOCTOR/PRACTITIONER:

_____

_____

_____

_____

_____

SUMMARY OF VISIT

RESULTS OF TESTING:

_____

_____

TESTING ORDERED FOR NEXT VISIT:

_____

_____

MEDICATION CHANGES:

_____

_____

REFERRALS:

_____

MEDICAL ONCOLOGY VISIT SUMMARY DATE: _____

DOCTOR/PRACTITIONER SEEN: _____

REASON FOR APPOINTMENT: _____

☐ NEW PATIENT VISIT   ☐ ROUTINE FOLLOWUP

☐ URGENT CARE VISIT   ☐ OTHER: _____

TESTING DONE FOR THIS APPOINTMENT: _____

_____

QUESTIONS FOR THE DOCTOR/PRACTITIONER: _____

_____

_____

_____

_____

SUMMARY OF VISIT

RESULTS OF TESTING: _____

_____

TESTING ORDERED FOR NEXT VISIT: _____

_____

MEDICATION CHANGES: _____

_____

REFERRALS: _____

MEDICAL ONCOLOGY VISIT SUMMARY DATE: _____

DOCTOR/PRACTITIONER SEEN:
_____

REASON FOR APPOINTMENT:
_____

☐ NEW PATIENT VISIT   ☐ ROUTINE FOLLOWUP

☐ URGENT CARE VISIT   ☐ OTHER:

TESTING DONE FOR THIS APPOINTMENT:
_____

_____

QUESTIONS FOR THE DOCTOR/PRACTITIONER:
_____

_____

_____

_____

SUMMARY OF VISIT

RESULTS OF TESTING:
_____

_____

TESTING ORDERED FOR NEXT VISIT:
_____

_____

MEDICATION CHANGES:
_____

_____

REFERRALS:
_____

MEDICAL ONCOLOGY VISIT SUMMARY DATE: _____

DOCTOR/PRACTITIONER SEEN: _____

REASON FOR APPOINTMENT: _____

☐ NEW PATIENT VISIT   ☐ ROUTINE FOLLOWUP _____

☐ URGENT CARE VISIT   ☐ OTHER: _____

TESTING DONE FOR THIS APPOINTMENT: _____

_____

QUESTIONS FOR THE DOCTOR/PRACTITIONER: _____

_____

_____

_____

_____

SUMMARY OF VISIT

RESULTS OF TESTING: _____

_____

TESTING ORDERED FOR NEXT VISIT: _____

_____

MEDICATION CHANGES: _____

_____

REFERRALS: _____

MEDICAL ONCOLOGY VISIT SUMMARY   DATE: _____

DOCTOR/PRACTITIONER SEEN:
_____

REASON FOR APPOINTMENT:
_____

☐ NEW PATIENT VISIT   ☐ ROUTINE FOLLOWUP

☐ URGENT CARE VISIT   ☐ OTHER:

TESTING DONE FOR THIS APPOINTMENT:
_____
_____

QUESTIONS FOR THE DOCTOR/PRACTITIONER:
_____
_____
_____
_____

SUMMARY OF VISIT

RESULTS OF TESTING:
_____
_____

TESTING ORDERED FOR NEXT VISIT:
_____
_____

MEDICATION CHANGES:
_____
_____

REFERRALS:
_____

MEDICAL ONCOLOGY VISIT SUMMARY DATE: _____

DOCTOR/PRACTITIONER SEEN: _____

REASON FOR APPOINTMENT: _____

☐ NEW PATIENT VISIT   ☐ ROUTINE FOLLOWUP

☐ URGENT CARE VISIT   ☐ OTHER: _____

TESTING DONE FOR THIS APPOINTMENT: _____
_____

QUESTIONS FOR THE DOCTOR/PRACTITIONER: _____
_____
_____
_____
_____

SUMMARY OF VISIT
_____

RESULTS OF TESTING: _____
_____

TESTING ORDERED FOR NEXT VISIT: _____
_____

MEDICATION CHANGES: _____
_____

REFERRALS: _____

MEDICAL ONCOLOGY VISIT SUMMARY DATE: _____

DOCTOR/PRACTITIONER SEEN:
_____

REASON FOR APPOINTMENT:
_____

☐ NEW PATIENT VISIT   ☐ ROUTINE FOLLOWUP

☐ URGENT CARE VISIT   ☐ OTHER:
_____

TESTING DONE FOR THIS APPOINTMENT:
_____
_____

QUESTIONS FOR THE DOCTOR/PRACTITIONER:
_____
_____
_____
_____
_____

SUMMARY OF VISIT
_____

RESULTS OF TESTING:
_____
_____

TESTING ORDERED FOR NEXT VISIT:
_____
_____

MEDICATION CHANGES:
_____
_____

REFERRALS:
_____

MEDICAL ONCOLOGY VISIT SUMMARY DATE: _____

DOCTOR/PRACTITIONER SEEN: _____

REASON FOR APPOINTMENT: _____

☐ NEW PATIENT VISIT   ☐ ROUTINE FOLLOWUP

☐ URGENT CARE VISIT   ☐ OTHER: _____

TESTING DONE FOR THIS APPOINTMENT:

_____

_____

QUESTIONS FOR THE DOCTOR/PRACTITIONER:

_____

_____

_____

_____

SUMMARY OF VISIT

RESULTS OF TESTING: _____

_____

TESTING ORDERED FOR NEXT VISIT: _____

_____

MEDICATION CHANGES: _____

_____

REFERRALS: _____

MEDICAL ONCOLOGY VISIT SUMMARY DATE: _____

DOCTOR/PRACTITIONER SEEN:
_____

REASON FOR APPOINTMENT:
_____

☐ NEW PATIENT VISIT   ☐ ROUTINE FOLLOWUP

☐ URGENT CARE VISIT   ☐ OTHER: _____

TESTING DONE FOR THIS APPOINTMENT:
_____
_____

QUESTIONS FOR THE DOCTOR/PRACTITIONER:
_____
_____
_____
_____

SUMMARY OF VISIT
_____

RESULTS OF TESTING:
_____
_____

TESTING ORDERED FOR NEXT VISIT:
_____
_____

MEDICATION CHANGES:
_____
_____

REFERRALS:
_____

MEDICAL ONCOLOGY VISIT SUMMARY DATE: _____

DOCTOR/PRACTITIONER SEEN: _____

REASON FOR APPOINTMENT: _____

☐ NEW PATIENT VISIT   ☐ ROUTINE FOLLOWUP

☐ URGENT CARE VISIT   ☐ OTHER:

TESTING DONE FOR THIS APPOINTMENT: _____

_____

QUESTIONS FOR THE DOCTOR/PRACTITIONER: _____

_____

_____

_____

_____

SUMMARY OF VISIT

RESULTS OF TESTING: _____

_____

TESTING ORDERED FOR NEXT VISIT: _____

_____

MEDICATION CHANGES: _____

_____

REFERRALS: _____

MEDICAL ONCOLOGY VISIT SUMMARY   DATE: _____

DOCTOR/PRACTITIONER SEEN:
_____

REASON FOR APPOINTMENT:
_____

☐ NEW PATIENT VISIT   ☐ ROUTINE FOLLOWUP

☐ URGENT CARE VISIT   ☐ OTHER:

TESTING DONE FOR THIS APPOINTMENT:
_____
_____

QUESTIONS FOR THE DOCTOR/PRACTITIONER:
_____
_____
_____
_____

SUMMARY OF VISIT

RESULTS OF TESTING:
_____
_____

TESTING ORDERED FOR NEXT VISIT:
_____
_____

MEDICATION CHANGES:
_____
_____

REFERRALS:
_____

MEDICAL ONCOLOGY VISIT SUMMARY DATE: _____

DOCTOR/PRACTITIONER SEEN: _____

REASON FOR APPOINTMENT: _____

☐ NEW PATIENT VISIT   ☐ ROUTINE FOLLOWUP

☐ URGENT CARE VISIT   ☐ OTHER: _____

TESTING DONE FOR THIS APPOINTMENT: _____

_____

QUESTIONS FOR THE DOCTOR/PRACTITIONER: _____

_____

_____

_____

_____

SUMMARY OF VISIT

RESULTS OF TESTING: _____

_____

TESTING ORDERED FOR NEXT VISIT: _____

_____

MEDICATION CHANGES: _____

_____

REFERRALS: _____

MEDICAL ONCOLOGY VISIT SUMMARY DATE: _____

DOCTOR/PRACTITIONER SEEN:
_____

REASON FOR APPOINTMENT:
_____

☐ NEW PATIENT VISIT   ☐ ROUTINE FOLLOWUP

☐ URGENT CARE VISIT   ☐ OTHER:
_____

TESTING DONE FOR THIS APPOINTMENT:
_____
_____

QUESTIONS FOR THE DOCTOR/PRACTITIONER:
_____
_____
_____
_____

SUMMARY OF VISIT

RESULTS OF TESTING:
_____
_____

TESTING ORDERED FOR NEXT VISIT:
_____
_____

MEDICATION CHANGES:
_____
_____

REFERRALS:
_____

MEDICAL ONCOLOGY VISIT SUMMARY DATE: _____

DOCTOR/PRACTITIONER SEEN: _____

REASON FOR APPOINTMENT: _____

☐ NEW PATIENT VISIT   ☐ ROUTINE FOLLOWUP _____

☐ URGENT CARE VISIT   ☐ OTHER: _____

TESTING DONE FOR THIS APPOINTMENT: _____

_____

QUESTIONS FOR THE DOCTOR/PRACTITIONER: _____

_____

_____

_____

_____

SUMMARY OF VISIT

RESULTS OF TESTING: _____

_____

TESTING ORDERED FOR NEXT VISIT: _____

_____

MEDICATION CHANGES: _____

_____

REFERRALS: _____

MEDICAL ONCOLOGY VISIT SUMMARY DATE: _____

DOCTOR/PRACTITIONER SEEN:
_____

REASON FOR APPOINTMENT:
_____

☐ NEW PATIENT VISIT   ☐ ROUTINE FOLLOWUP

☐ URGENT CARE VISIT   ☐ OTHER:

TESTING DONE FOR THIS APPOINTMENT:
_____
_____

QUESTIONS FOR THE DOCTOR/PRACTITIONER:
_____
_____
_____
_____

SUMMARY OF VISIT

RESULTS OF TESTING:
_____
_____

TESTING ORDERED FOR NEXT VISIT:
_____
_____

MEDICATION CHANGES:
_____
_____

REFERRALS:
_____

MEDICAL ONCOLOGY VISIT SUMMARY DATE: _____

DOCTOR/PRACTITIONER SEEN: _____

REASON FOR APPOINTMENT: _____

☐ NEW PATIENT VISIT   ☐ ROUTINE FOLLOWUP

☐ URGENT CARE VISIT   ☐ OTHER: _____

TESTING DONE FOR THIS APPOINTMENT:
_____
_____

QUESTIONS FOR THE DOCTOR/PRACTITIONER:
_____
_____
_____
_____

SUMMARY OF VISIT

RESULTS OF TESTING:
_____
_____

TESTING ORDERED FOR NEXT VISIT:
_____
_____

MEDICATION CHANGES:
_____
_____

REFERRALS:
_____

MEDICAL ONCOLOGY VISIT SUMMARY DATE: _____

DOCTOR/PRACTITIONER SEEN:
_____

REASON FOR APPOINTMENT:
_____

☐ NEW PATIENT VISIT   ☐ ROUTINE FOLLOWUP

☐ URGENT CARE VISIT   ☐ OTHER: _____

TESTING DONE FOR THIS APPOINTMENT:
_____
_____

QUESTIONS FOR THE DOCTOR/PRACTITIONER:
_____
_____
_____
_____

SUMMARY OF VISIT

RESULTS OF TESTING:
_____
_____

TESTING ORDERED FOR NEXT VISIT:
_____
_____

MEDICATION CHANGES:
_____
_____

REFERRALS:
_____

MEDICAL ONCOLOGY VISIT SUMMARY DATE: _____

DOCTOR/PRACTITIONER SEEN: _____

REASON FOR APPOINTMENT: _____

☐ NEW PATIENT VISIT   ☐ ROUTINE FOLLOWUP

☐ URGENT CARE VISIT   ☐ OTHER: _____

TESTING DONE FOR THIS APPOINTMENT: _____

_____

QUESTIONS FOR THE DOCTOR/PRACTITIONER: _____

_____

_____

_____

_____

SUMMARY OF VISIT

RESULTS OF TESTING: _____

_____

TESTING ORDERED FOR NEXT VISIT: _____

_____

MEDICATION CHANGES: _____

_____

REFERRALS: _____

NOTES

NOTES

CHEMOTHERAPY, IMMUNOTHERAPY AND OTHER CANCER MEDICATIONS

CHEMOTHERAPY, IMMUNOTHERAPY AND OTHER CANCER MEDICATIONS LOG

TYPE OF THERAPY:

☐ INTRAVENOUS (BY VEIN)

☐ ORAL (BY MOUTH) IF YES TO ORAL MEDICATION, SKIP THE INFUSION SECTION AND GO TO THE ORAL MEDICATION FOR CANCER SECTION

☐ INTRAMUSCULAR (SHOT)

☐ SUBCUTANEOUS (SHOT)

☐ OTHER:

INFUSION SECTION:

INFUSION CYCLE:

DATE:

DRUG 1:   DOSE:

DRUG 2:   DOSE:

DRUG 3:   DOSE:

DRUG 4:   DOSE:

CYCLES ANTICIPATED:

NOTES:

INFUSION SECTION:

INFUSION CYCLE:
_____

DATE:
_____

DRUG 1: _____ DOSE: _____

DRUG 2: _____ DOSE: _____

DRUG 3: _____ DOSE: _____

DRUG 4: _____ DOSE: _____

CYCLES ANTICIPATED:
_____

NOTES:
_____
_____

INFUSION SECTION:

INFUSION CYCLE:
_____

DATE:
_____

DRUG 1: _____ DOSE: _____

DRUG 2: _____ DOSE: _____

DRUG 3: _____ DOSE: _____

DRUG 4: _____ DOSE: _____

CYCLES ANTICIPATED:
_____

NOTES:
_____

INFUSION SECTION:

INFUSION CYCLE:
_____

DATE:
_____

DRUG 1: _____ DOSE: _____

DRUG 2: _____ DOSE: _____

DRUG 3: _____ DOSE: _____

DRUG 4: _____ DOSE: _____

CYCLES ANTICIPATED:
_____

NOTES:
_____

_____

INFUSION SECTION:

INFUSION CYCLE:
_____

DATE:
_____

DRUG 1: _____ DOSE: _____

DRUG 2: _____ DOSE: _____

DRUG 3: _____ DOSE: _____

DRUG 4: _____ DOSE: _____

CYCLES ANTICIPATED:
_____

NOTES:
_____

ORAL MEDICATION:

NAME: _____   GENERIC NAME: _____

STRENGTH: _____   DOSE: _____

DIRECTIONS FOR TAKING MEDICATION: _____

_____

HOW MUCH SHOULD I TAKE?: _____

HOW OFTEN DO I TAKE IT?: _____

WHEN SHOULD I TAKE IT?: _____

SHOULD I TAKE IT: _____

☐ WITH WATER   ☐ WITH FOOD   ☐ WITHOUT FOOD

☐ MEAL TIMING IS NOT NECESSARY

ARE THERE SPECIFIC FOODS TO AVOID WHILE TAKING THIS MEDICINE?

_____

_____

ARE THERE BEVERAGES TO AVOID WHILE TAKING THIS MEDICINE?

_____

_____

IS IT SAFE TO TAKE WITH OTHER MEDICATIONS?

☐ YES   ☐ NO   AVOID: _____

_____

START DATE: _____

HOW DO I STORE THE DRUG?

☐ ROOM TEMPERATURE ☐ REFRIGERATOR ☐ AVOID SUNLIGHT

☐ OTHER:

ARE THERE PRECAUTIONS THAT MY FAMILY MEMBERS HAVE TO TAKE?

☐ NO ☐ YES:

THREE MOST COMMON SIDE EFFECTS TO WATCH FOR:

1.)

2.)

3.)

HAVE I MISSED ANY DOSES? ☐ YES ☐ NO

DATES OF MISSED DOSES:

WHAT SHOULD I DO WHEN I REALIZE THAT I MISSED A DOSE?

☐ CALL THE DOCTOR'S OFFICE AND SPEAK WITH THE ON-CALL DOCTOR

☐ DON'T "CATCH UP". JUST TAKE YOUR NEXT SCHEDULED DOSE

HOW OFTEN DO I NEED BLOOD WORK?

END DATE:

ORAL MEDICATION:

NAME: _____ GENERIC NAME: _____

STRENGTH: _____ DOSE: _____

DIRECTIONS FOR TAKING MEDICATION: _____

_____

HOW MUCH SHOULD I TAKE?: _____

HOW OFTEN DO I TAKE IT?: _____

WHEN SHOULD I TAKE IT?: _____

SHOULD I TAKE IT: _____

☐ WITH WATER ☐ WITH FOOD ☐ WITHOUT FOOD

☐ MEAL TIMING IS NOT NECESSARY

ARE THERE SPECIFIC FOODS TO AVOID WHILE TAKING THIS MEDICINE?

_____

_____

ARE THERE BEVERAGES TO AVOID WHILE TAKING THIS MEDICINE?

_____

_____

IS IT SAFE TO TAKE WITH OTHER MEDICATIONS?

☐ YES   ☐ NO   AVOID: _____

_____

_____

START DATE: _____

HOW DO I STORE THE DRUG?

☐ ROOM TEMPERATURE   ☐ REFRIGERATOR   ☐ AVOID SUNLIGHT

☐ OTHER:

ARE THERE PRECAUTIONS THAT MY FAMILY MEMBERS HAVE TO TAKE?

☐ NO   ☐ YES:

THREE MOST COMMON SIDE EFFECTS TO WATCH FOR:

1.)

2.)

3.)

HAVE I MISSED ANY DOSES? ☐ YES   ☐ NO

DATES OF MISSED DOSES:

WHAT SHOULD I DO WHEN I REALIZE THAT I MISSED A DOSE?

☐ CALL THE DOCTOR'S OFFICE AND SPEAK WITH THE ON-CALL DOCTOR

☐ DON'T "CATCH UP". JUST TAKE YOUR NEXT SCHEDULED DOSE

HOW OFTEN DO I NEED BLOOD WORK?

END DATE:

ORAL MEDICATION:

NAME: _____   GENERIC NAME: _____

STRENGTH: _____   DOSE: _____

DIRECTIONS FOR TAKING MEDICATION: _____

_____

HOW MUCH SHOULD I TAKE?: _____

HOW OFTEN DO I TAKE IT?: _____

WHEN SHOULD I TAKE IT?: _____

SHOULD I TAKE IT: _____

☐ WITH WATER   ☐ WITH FOOD   ☐ WITHOUT FOOD

☐ MEAL TIMING IS NOT NECESSARY

ARE THERE SPECIFIC FOODS TO AVOID WHILE TAKING THIS MEDICINE?

_____

ARE THERE BEVERAGES TO AVOID WHILE TAKING THIS MEDICINE?

_____

IS IT SAFE TO TAKE WITH OTHER MEDICATIONS?

☐ YES   ☐ NO   AVOID: _____

_____

START DATE: _____

HOW DO I STORE THE DRUG?

☐ ROOM TEMPERATURE ☐ REFRIGERATOR ☐ AVOID SUNLIGHT

☐ OTHER:

ARE THERE PRECAUTIONS THAT MY FAMILY MEMBERS HAVE TO TAKE?

☐ NO ☐ YES:

THREE MOST COMMON SIDE EFFECTS TO WATCH FOR:

1.)

2.)

3.)

HAVE I MISSED ANY DOSES? ☐ YES ☐ NO

DATES OF MISSED DOSES:

WHAT SHOULD I DO WHEN I REALIZE THAT I MISSED A DOSE?

☐ CALL THE DOCTOR'S OFFICE AND SPEAK WITH THE ON-CALL DOCTOR

☐ DON'T "CATCH UP". JUST TAKE YOUR NEXT SCHEDULED DOSE

HOW OFTEN DO I NEED BLOOD WORK?

END DATE:

WEEK 1		SUN	MON	TUES	WED	THURS	FRI	SAT
	DATE:							
ANTINAUSEA	AM							
	PM							
CANCER MEDICATION	AM							
	PM							

WEEK 2		SUN	MON	TUES	WED	THURS	FRI	SAT
	DATE:							
ANTINAUSEA	AM							
	PM							
CANCER MEDICATION	AM							
	PM							

WEEK 3		SUN	MON	TUES	WED	THURS	FRI	SAT
	DATE:							
ANTINAUSEA	AM							
	PM							
CANCER MEDICATION	AM							
	PM							

WEEK 4		SUN	MON	TUES	WED	THURS	FRI	SAT
	DATE:							
ANTINAUSEA	AM							
	PM							
CANCER MEDICATION	AM							
	PM							

WEEK 1		SUN	MON	TUES	WED	THURS	FRI	SAT
	DATE:							
ANTINAUSEA	AM							
	PM							
CANCER MEDICATION	AM							
	PM							

WEEK 2		SUN	MON	TUES	WED	THURS	FRI	SAT
	DATE:							
ANTINAUSEA	AM							
	PM							
CANCER MEDICATION	AM							
	PM							

WEEK 3		SUN	MON	TUES	WED	THURS	FRI	SAT
	DATE:							
ANTINAUSEA	AM							
	PM							
CANCER MEDICATION	AM							
	PM							

WEEK 4		SUN	MON	TUES	WED	THURS	FRI	SAT
	DATE:							
ANTINAUSEA	AM							
	PM							
CANCER MEDICATION	AM							
	PM							

WEEK 1		SUN	MON	TUES	WED	THURS	FRI	SAT
	DATE:							
ANTINAUSEA	AM							
	PM							
CANCER MEDICATION	AM							
	PM							

WEEK 2		SUN	MON	TUES	WED	THURS	FRI	SAT
	DATE:							
ANTINAUSEA	AM							
	PM							
CANCER MEDICATION	AM							
	PM							

WEEK 3		SUN	MON	TUES	WED	THURS	FRI	SAT
	DATE:							
ANTINAUSEA	AM							
	PM							
CANCER MEDICATION	AM							
	PM							

WEEK 4		SUN	MON	TUES	WED	THURS	FRI	SAT
	DATE:							
ANTINAUSEA	AM							
	PM							
CANCER MEDICATION	AM							
	PM							

WEEK 1		SUN	MON	TUES	WED	THURS	FRI	SAT
	DATE:							
ANTINAUSEA	AM							
	PM							
CANCER MEDICATION	AM							
	PM							

WEEK 2		SUN	MON	TUES	WED	THURS	FRI	SAT
	DATE:							
ANTINAUSEA	AM							
	PM							
CANCER MEDICATION	AM							
	PM							

WEEK 3		SUN	MON	TUES	WED	THURS	FRI	SAT
	DATE:							
ANTINAUSEA	AM							
	PM							
CANCER MEDICATION	AM							
	PM							

WEEK 4		SUN	MON	TUES	WED	THURS	FRI	SAT
	DATE:							
ANTINAUSEA	AM							
	PM							
CANCER MEDICATION	AM							
	PM							

WEEK 1		SUN	MON	TUES	WED	THURS	FRI	SAT
	DATE:							
ANTINAUSEA	AM							
	PM							
CANCER MEDICATION	AM							
	PM							

WEEK 2		SUN	MON	TUES	WED	THURS	FRI	SAT
	DATE:							
ANTINAUSEA	AM							
	PM							
CANCER MEDICATION	AM							
	PM							

WEEK 3		SUN	MON	TUES	WED	THURS	FRI	SAT
	DATE:							
ANTINAUSEA	AM							
	PM							
CANCER MEDICATION	AM							
	PM							

WEEK 4		SUN	MON	TUES	WED	THURS	FRI	SAT
	DATE:							
ANTINAUSEA	AM							
	PM							
CANCER MEDICATION	AM							
	PM							

WEEK 1		SUN	MON	TUES	WED	THURS	FRI	SAT
	DATE:							
ANTINAUSEA	AM							
	PM							
CANCER MEDICATION	AM							
	PM							

WEEK 2		SUN	MON	TUES	WED	THURS	FRI	SAT
	DATE:							
ANTINAUSEA	AM							
	PM							
CANCER MEDICATION	AM							
	PM							

WEEK 3			SUN	MON	TUES	WED	THURS	FRI	SAT
	DATE:								
ANTINAUSEA	AM								
	PM								
CANCER MEDICATION	AM								
	PM								

WEEK 4			SUN	MON	TUES	WED	THURS	FRI	SAT
	DATE:								
ANTINAUSEA	AM								
	PM								
CANCER MEDICATION	AM								
	PM								

WEEK 1		SUN	MON	TUES	WED	THURS	FRI	SAT
	DATE:							
ANTINAUSEA	AM							
	PM							
CANCER MEDICATION	AM							
	PM							

WEEK 2		SUN	MON	TUES	WED	THURS	FRI	SAT
	DATE:							
ANTINAUSEA	AM							
	PM							
CANCER MEDICATION	AM							
	PM							

WEEK 3		SUN	MON	TUES	WED	THURS	FRI	SAT
	DATE:							
ANTINAUSEA	AM							
	PM							
CANCER MEDICATION	AM							
	PM							

WEEK 4		SUN	MON	TUES	WED	THURS	FRI	SAT
	DATE:							
ANTINAUSEA	AM							
	PM							
CANCER MEDICATION	AM							
	PM							

WEEK 1		SUN	MON	TUES	WED	THURS	FRI	SAT
	DATE:							
ANTINAUSEA	AM							
	PM							
CANCER MEDICATION	AM							
	PM							

WEEK 2		SUN	MON	TUES	WED	THURS	FRI	SAT
	DATE:							
ANTINAUSEA	AM							
	PM							
CANCER MEDICATION	AM							
	PM							

WEEK 3		SUN	MON	TUES	WED	THURS	FRI	SAT
	DATE:							
ANTINAUSEA	AM							
	PM							
CANCER MEDICATION	AM							
	PM							

WEEK 4		SUN	MON	TUES	WED	THURS	FRI	SAT
	DATE:							
ANTINAUSEA	AM							
	PM							
CANCER MEDICATION	AM							
	PM							

WEEK 1		SUN	MON	TUES	WED	THURS	FRI	SAT
	DATE:							
ANTINAUSEA	AM							
	PM							
CANCER MEDICATION	AM							
	PM							

WEEK 2		SUN	MON	TUES	WED	THURS	FRI	SAT
	DATE:							
ANTINAUSEA	AM							
	PM							
CANCER MEDICATION	AM							
	PM							

WEEK 3		SUN	MON	TUES	WED	THURS	FRI	SAT
	DATE:							
ANTINAUSEA	AM							
	PM							
CANCER MEDICATION	AM							
	PM							

WEEK 4		SUN	MON	TUES	WED	THURS	FRI	SAT
	DATE:							
ANTINAUSEA	AM							
	PM							
CANCER MEDICATION	AM							
	PM							

WEEK 1		SUN	MON	TUES	WED	THURS	FRI	SAT
	DATE:							
ANTINAUSEA	AM							
	PM							
CANCER MEDICATION	AM							
	PM							

WEEK 2		SUN	MON	TUES	WED	THURS	FRI	SAT
	DATE:							
ANTINAUSEA	AM							
	PM							
CANCER MEDICATION	AM							
	PM							

WEEK 3		SUN	MON	TUES	WED	THURS	FRI	SAT
	DATE:							
ANTINAUSEA	AM							
	PM							
CANCER MEDICATION	AM							
	PM							

WEEK 4		SUN	MON	TUES	WED	THURS	FRI	SAT
	DATE:							
ANTINAUSEA	AM							
	PM							
CANCER MEDICATION	AM							
	PM							

WEEK 1		SUN	MON	TUES	WED	THURS	FRI	SAT
	DATE:							
ANTINAUSEA	AM							
	PM							
CANCER MEDICATION	AM							
	PM							

WEEK 2		SUN	MON	TUES	WED	THURS	FRI	SAT
	DATE:							
ANTINAUSEA	AM							
	PM							
CANCER MEDICATION	AM							
	PM							

WEEK 3		SUN	MON	TUES	WED	THURS	FRI	SAT
	DATE:							
ANTINAUSEA	AM							
	PM							
CANCER MEDICATION	AM							
	PM							

WEEK 4		SUN	MON	TUES	WED	THURS	FRI	SAT
	DATE:							
ANTINAUSEA	AM							
	PM							
CANCER MEDICATION	AM							
	PM							

WEEK 1			SUN	MON	TUES	WED	THURS	FRI	SAT
		DATE:							
ANTINAUSEA		AM							
		PM							
CANCER MEDICATION		AM							
		PM							

WEEK 2			SUN	MON	TUES	WED	THURS	FRI	SAT
		DATE:							
ANTINAUSEA		AM							
		PM							
CANCER MEDICATION		AM							
		PM							

WEEK 3		SUN	MON	TUES	WED	THURS	FRI	SAT
	DATE:							
ANTINAUSEA	AM							
	PM							
CANCER MEDICATION	AM							
	PM							

WEEK 4		SUN	MON	TUES	WED	THURS	FRI	SAT
	DATE:							
ANTINAUSEA	AM							
	PM							
CANCER MEDICATION	AM							
	PM							

OTHER MEDICATION LOG

MEDICATION NAME:

REASON:

START DATE:

END DATE:

DOSE:

NOTES:

MEDICATION NAME:

REASON:

START DATE:

END DATE:

DOSE:

NOTES:

MEDICATION NAME: _____

REASON: _____

START DATE: _____

END DATE: _____

DOSE: _____

_____

NOTES: _____

_____

_____

MEDICATION NAME: _____

REASON: _____

START DATE: _____

END DATE: _____

DOSE: _____

_____

NOTES: _____

_____

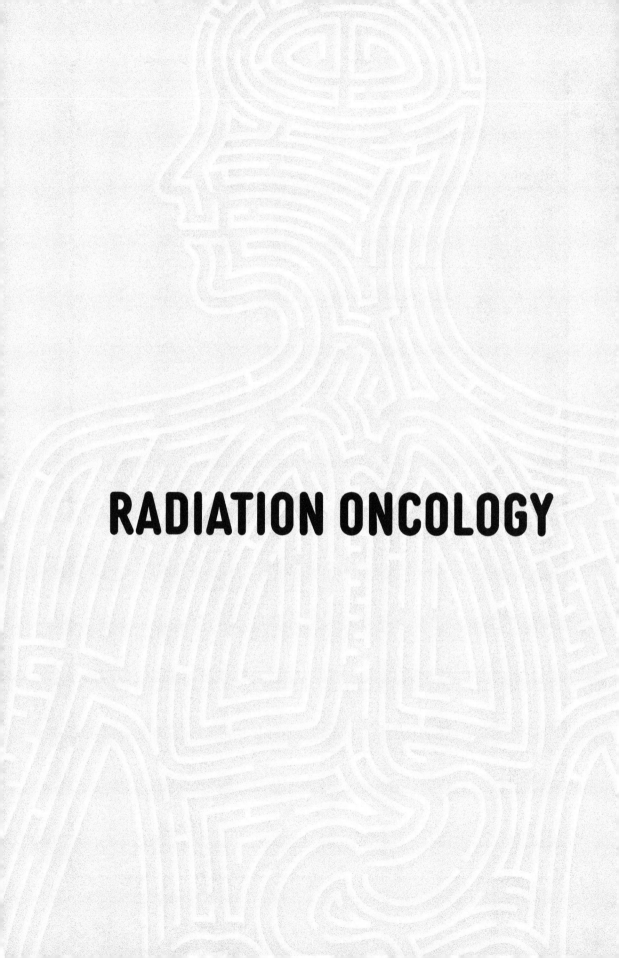

RADIATION ONCOLOGY

MY RADIATION TEAM

NAME OF RADIATION PRACTICE: _____

_____

ADDRESS: _____ PHONE: _____

_____

PHYSICIAN: _____ PHONE: _____

_____

NURSE PRACTITIONER: _____ PHONE: _____

_____

PHYSICIAN ASSISTANT: _____ PHONE: _____

_____

NURSE/NURSE NAVIGATOR: _____ PHONE: _____

_____

SCHEDULER: _____ PHONE: _____

_____

PATIENT PORTAL WEBSITE ADDRESS: _____

_____

ADDITIONAL INFO: _____

_____

MY RADIATION TREATMENT PLAN

Show this page to your Radiation Oncologist and ask them to tell you which type of radiation therapy you will have.

☐ EXTERNAL BEAM RADIATION: _____

TYPE: _____

☐ STEREOTACTIC RADIATION (SRS) _____

TYPE: _____

☐ INTERNAL BEAM RADIATION: _____

TYPE: _____

☐ BRACHYTHERAPY: _____

☐ OTHER: _____

NUMBER OF TREATMENTS PLANNED: _____

NUMBER OF TREATMENTS RECEIVED: _____

BODY LOCATION THAT WAS TREATED: _____

_____

START DATE: _____

END DATE: _____

_____

SIDE EFFECTS: _____

MY RADIATION TREATMENT PLAN

Show this page to your Radiation Oncologist and ask them to tell you which type of radiation therapy you will have.

☐ EXTERNAL BEAM RADIATION: _____

TYPE: _____

☐ STEREOTACTIC RADIATION (SRS) _____

TYPE: _____

☐ INTERNAL BEAM RADIATION: _____

TYPE: _____

☐ BRACHYTHERAPY: _____

☐ OTHER: _____

NUMBER OF TREATMENTS PLANNED: _____

NUMBER OF TREATMENTS RECEIVED: _____

BODY LOCATION THAT WAS TREATED: _____

_____

START DATE: _____

END DATE: _____

_____

SIDE EFFECTS: _____

MY RADIATION TREATMENT PLAN

Show this page to your Radiation Oncologist and ask them to tell you which type of radiation therapy you will have.

☐ EXTERNAL BEAM RADIATION:
_____

TYPE:
_____

☐ STEREOTACTIC RADIATION (SRS)
_____

TYPE:
_____

☐ INTERNAL BEAM RADIATION:
_____

TYPE:
_____

☐ BRACHYTHERAPY:
_____

☐ OTHER:
_____

NUMBER OF TREATMENTS PLANNED:
_____

NUMBER OF TREATMENTS RECEIVED:
_____

BODY LOCATION THAT WAS TREATED:
_____

_____

START DATE:
_____

END DATE:
_____

_____

SIDE EFFECTS:
_____

MY RADIATION TREATMENT PLAN

Show this page to your Radiation Oncologist and ask them to tell you which type of radiation therapy you will have.

☐ EXTERNAL BEAM RADIATION: _____

TYPE: _____

☐ STEREOTACTIC RADIATION (SRS) _____

TYPE: _____

☐ INTERNAL BEAM RADIATION: _____

TYPE: _____

☐ BRACHYTHERAPY: _____

☐ OTHER: _____

NUMBER OF TREATMENTS PLANNED: _____

NUMBER OF TREATMENTS RECEIVED: _____

BODY LOCATION THAT WAS TREATED: _____

_____

START DATE: _____

END DATE: _____

_____

SIDE EFFECTS: _____

RADIATION VISIT SUMMARY   DATE: _____

DOCTOR/PRACTITIONER SEEN:
_____

REASON FOR APPOINTMENT:
_____

☐ PRE TREATMENT VISIT   ☐ WEEKLY TREATMENT VISIT

☐ POST TREATMENT VISIT   ☐ OTHER: _____

TESTING DONE FOR THIS APPOINTMENT:
_____
_____

QUESTIONS FOR THE DOCTOR/PRACTITIONER:
_____
_____
_____
_____
_____

SUMMARY OF VISIT

RESULTS OF TESTING:
_____
_____

TESTING ORDERED FOR NEXT VISIT:
_____
_____

MEDICATION CHANGES:
_____
_____

REFERRALS:
_____

RADIATION VISIT SUMMARY   DATE: _____

DOCTOR/PRACTITIONER SEEN: _____

REASON FOR APPOINTMENT: _____

☐ PRE TREATMENT VISIT   ☐ WEEKLY TREATMENT VISIT

☐ POST TREATMENT VISIT   ☐ OTHER: _____

TESTING DONE FOR THIS APPOINTMENT:
_____
_____

QUESTIONS FOR THE DOCTOR/PRACTITIONER:
_____
_____
_____
_____

SUMMARY OF VISIT

RESULTS OF TESTING:
_____
_____

TESTING ORDERED FOR NEXT VISIT:
_____
_____

MEDICATION CHANGES:
_____
_____

REFERRALS:
_____

RADIATION VISIT SUMMARY

DATE: _____

DOCTOR/PRACTITIONER SEEN: _____

REASON FOR APPOINTMENT: _____

☐ PRE TREATMENT VISIT   ☐ WEEKLY TREATMENT VISIT

☐ POST TREATMENT VISIT   ☐ OTHER: _____

TESTING DONE FOR THIS APPOINTMENT:

_____

_____

QUESTIONS FOR THE DOCTOR/PRACTITIONER:

_____

_____

_____

_____

SUMMARY OF VISIT

RESULTS OF TESTING:

_____

_____

TESTING ORDERED FOR NEXT VISIT:

_____

_____

MEDICATION CHANGES:

_____

_____

REFERRALS:

_____

RADIATION VISIT SUMMARY   DATE: _____

DOCTOR/PRACTITIONER SEEN: _____

REASON FOR APPOINTMENT: _____

☐ PRE TREATMENT VISIT   ☐ WEEKLY TREATMENT VISIT

☐ POST TREATMENT VISIT   ☐ OTHER: _____

TESTING DONE FOR THIS APPOINTMENT:
_____
_____

QUESTIONS FOR THE DOCTOR/PRACTITIONER:
_____
_____
_____
_____

SUMMARY OF VISIT

RESULTS OF TESTING: _____
_____

TESTING ORDERED FOR NEXT VISIT: _____
_____

MEDICATION CHANGES: _____
_____

REFERRALS: _____

RADIATION VISIT SUMMARY   DATE: _____

DOCTOR/PRACTITIONER SEEN: _____

REASON FOR APPOINTMENT: _____

☐ PRE TREATMENT VISIT   ☐ WEEKLY TREATMENT VISIT

☐ POST TREATMENT VISIT   ☐ OTHER: _____

TESTING DONE FOR THIS APPOINTMENT: _____
_____

QUESTIONS FOR THE DOCTOR/PRACTITIONER: _____
_____
_____
_____
_____

SUMMARY OF VISIT

RESULTS OF TESTING: _____
_____

TESTING ORDERED FOR NEXT VISIT: _____
_____

MEDICATION CHANGES: _____
_____

REFERRALS: _____

RADIATION VISIT SUMMARY   DATE: _____

DOCTOR/PRACTITIONER SEEN: _____

REASON FOR APPOINTMENT: _____

☐ PRE TREATMENT VISIT   ☐ WEEKLY TREATMENT VISIT

☐ POST TREATMENT VISIT   ☐ OTHER: _____

TESTING DONE FOR THIS APPOINTMENT: _____

_____

QUESTIONS FOR THE DOCTOR/PRACTITIONER: _____

_____

_____

_____

_____

SUMMARY OF VISIT

RESULTS OF TESTING: _____

_____

TESTING ORDERED FOR NEXT VISIT: _____

_____

MEDICATION CHANGES: _____

_____

REFERRALS: _____

RADIATION VISIT SUMMARY   DATE: _____

DOCTOR/PRACTITIONER SEEN: _____

REASON FOR APPOINTMENT: _____

☐ PRE TREATMENT VISIT   ☐ WEEKLY TREATMENT VISIT

☐ POST TREATMENT VISIT   ☐ OTHER: _____

TESTING DONE FOR THIS APPOINTMENT:
_____
_____

QUESTIONS FOR THE DOCTOR/PRACTITIONER:
_____
_____
_____
_____
_____

SUMMARY OF VISIT

RESULTS OF TESTING:
_____
_____

TESTING ORDERED FOR NEXT VISIT:
_____
_____

MEDICATION CHANGES:
_____
_____

REFERRALS:
_____

RADIATION VISIT SUMMARY   DATE: _____

DOCTOR/PRACTITIONER SEEN: _____

REASON FOR APPOINTMENT: _____

☐ PRE TREATMENT VISIT   ☐ WEEKLY TREATMENT VISIT

☐ POST TREATMENT VISIT   ☐ OTHER: _____

TESTING DONE FOR THIS APPOINTMENT:
_____
_____

QUESTIONS FOR THE DOCTOR/PRACTITIONER:
_____
_____
_____
_____

SUMMARY OF VISIT

RESULTS OF TESTING:
_____
_____

TESTING ORDERED FOR NEXT VISIT:
_____
_____

MEDICATION CHANGES:
_____
_____

REFERRALS:
_____

RADIATION VISIT SUMMARY   DATE: _____

DOCTOR/PRACTITIONER SEEN:
_____

REASON FOR APPOINTMENT:
_____

☐ PRE TREATMENT VISIT   ☐ WEEKLY TREATMENT VISIT

☐ POST TREATMENT VISIT   ☐ OTHER: _____

TESTING DONE FOR THIS APPOINTMENT:
_____
_____

QUESTIONS FOR THE DOCTOR/PRACTITIONER:
_____
_____
_____
_____
_____

SUMMARY OF VISIT

RESULTS OF TESTING:
_____
_____

TESTING ORDERED FOR NEXT VISIT:
_____
_____

MEDICATION CHANGES:
_____
_____

REFERRALS:
_____

RADIATION VISIT SUMMARY   DATE: _____

DOCTOR/PRACTITIONER SEEN: _____

REASON FOR APPOINTMENT: _____

☐ PRE TREATMENT VISIT   ☐ WEEKLY TREATMENT VISIT

☐ POST TREATMENT VISIT   ☐ OTHER: _____

TESTING DONE FOR THIS APPOINTMENT: _____

_____

QUESTIONS FOR THE DOCTOR/PRACTITIONER: _____

_____

_____

_____

_____

SUMMARY OF VISIT

RESULTS OF TESTING: _____

_____

TESTING ORDERED FOR NEXT VISIT: _____

_____

MEDICATION CHANGES: _____

_____

REFERRALS: _____

RADIATION VISIT SUMMARY

DATE: _____

DOCTOR/PRACTITIONER SEEN:
_____

REASON FOR APPOINTMENT:
_____

☐ PRE TREATMENT VISIT   ☐ WEEKLY TREATMENT VISIT

☐ POST TREATMENT VISIT   ☐ OTHER:

TESTING DONE FOR THIS APPOINTMENT:
_____
_____

QUESTIONS FOR THE DOCTOR/PRACTITIONER:
_____
_____
_____
_____

SUMMARY OF VISIT

RESULTS OF TESTING:
_____
_____

TESTING ORDERED FOR NEXT VISIT:
_____
_____

MEDICATION CHANGES:
_____
_____

REFERRALS:
_____

RADIATION VISIT SUMMARY   DATE: _____

DOCTOR/PRACTITIONER SEEN: _____

REASON FOR APPOINTMENT: _____

☐ PRE TREATMENT VISIT   ☐ WEEKLY TREATMENT VISIT

☐ POST TREATMENT VISIT   ☐ OTHER: _____

TESTING DONE FOR THIS APPOINTMENT:
_____
_____

QUESTIONS FOR THE DOCTOR/PRACTITIONER:
_____
_____
_____
_____
_____

SUMMARY OF VISIT

RESULTS OF TESTING:
_____
_____

TESTING ORDERED FOR NEXT VISIT:
_____
_____

MEDICATION CHANGES:
_____
_____

REFERRALS:
_____

RADIATION VISIT SUMMARY

DATE: _____

DOCTOR/PRACTITIONER SEEN:
_____

REASON FOR APPOINTMENT:
_____

☐ PRE TREATMENT VISIT   ☐ WEEKLY TREATMENT VISIT

☐ POST TREATMENT VISIT   ☐ OTHER:

TESTING DONE FOR THIS APPOINTMENT:
_____
_____

QUESTIONS FOR THE DOCTOR/PRACTITIONER:
_____
_____
_____
_____

SUMMARY OF VISIT

RESULTS OF TESTING:
_____
_____

TESTING ORDERED FOR NEXT VISIT:
_____
_____

MEDICATION CHANGES:
_____
_____

REFERRALS:
_____

RADIATION VISIT SUMMARY   DATE: _____

DOCTOR/PRACTITIONER SEEN: _____

REASON FOR APPOINTMENT: _____

☐ PRE TREATMENT VISIT   ☐ WEEKLY TREATMENT VISIT

☐ POST TREATMENT VISIT   ☐ OTHER: _____

TESTING DONE FOR THIS APPOINTMENT: _____

_____

QUESTIONS FOR THE DOCTOR/PRACTITIONER: _____

_____

_____

_____

_____

SUMMARY OF VISIT

RESULTS OF TESTING: _____

_____

TESTING ORDERED FOR NEXT VISIT: _____

_____

MEDICATION CHANGES: _____

_____

REFERRALS: _____

RADIATION VISIT SUMMARY   DATE: _____

DOCTOR/PRACTITIONER SEEN: _____

REASON FOR APPOINTMENT: _____

☐ PRE TREATMENT VISIT   ☐ WEEKLY TREATMENT VISIT

☐ POST TREATMENT VISIT   ☐ OTHER: _____

TESTING DONE FOR THIS APPOINTMENT:
_____
_____

QUESTIONS FOR THE DOCTOR/PRACTITIONER:
_____
_____
_____
_____
_____

SUMMARY OF VISIT

RESULTS OF TESTING:
_____
_____

TESTING ORDERED FOR NEXT VISIT:
_____
_____

MEDICATION CHANGES:
_____
_____

REFERRALS:
_____

NOTES

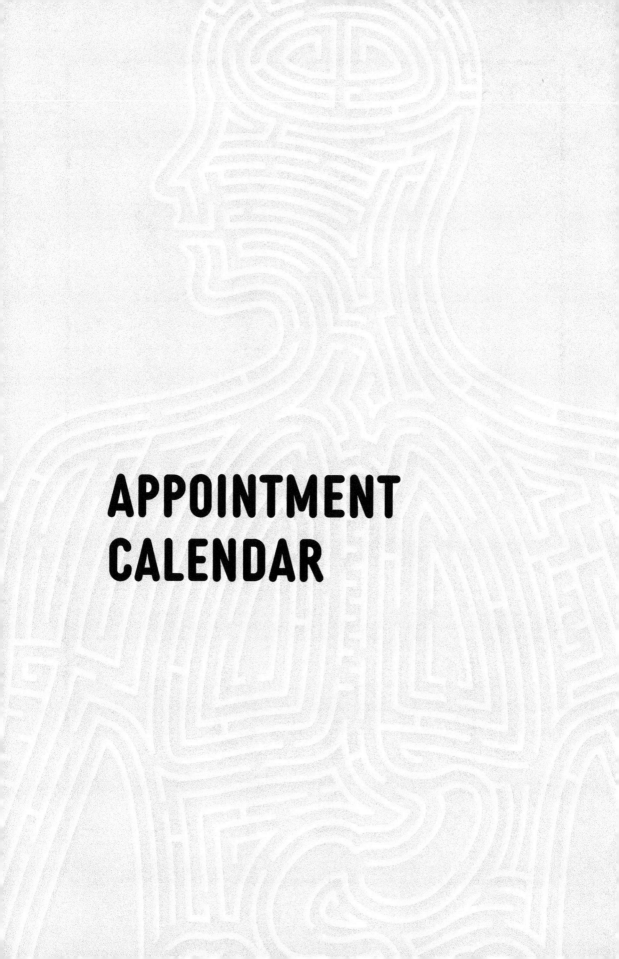

APPOINTMENT
CALENDAR

MON. DATE:	TUES. DATE:	WED. DATE:
THURS. DATE:	FRI. DATE:	SAT. DATE:
		SUN. DATE:

MON. DATE:	TUES. DATE:	WED. DATE:
THURS. DATE:	FRI. DATE:	SAT. DATE:
		SUN. DATE:

MON. DATE:	TUES. DATE:	WED. DATE:

THURS. DATE:	FRI. DATE:	SAT. DATE:
		SUN. DATE:

MON. DATE:	TUES. DATE:	WED. DATE:

THURS. DATE:	FRI. DATE:	SAT. DATE:
		SUN. DATE:

MON. DATE:	**TUES.** DATE:	**WED.** DATE:
THURS. DATE:	**FRI.** DATE:	**SAT.** DATE:
		SUN. DATE:

MON. DATE:	**TUES.** DATE:	**WED.** DATE:
THURS. DATE:	**FRI.** DATE:	**SAT.** DATE:
		SUN. DATE:

MON. DATE:	TUES. DATE:	WED. DATE:
THURS. DATE:	FRI. DATE:	SAT. DATE:
		SUN. DATE:

MON. DATE:	TUES. DATE:	WED. DATE:
THURS. DATE:	FRI. DATE:	SAT. DATE:
		SUN. DATE:

MON. DATE:	TUES. DATE:	WED. DATE:
THURS. DATE:	FRI. DATE:	SAT. DATE:
		SUN. DATE:

MON. DATE:	TUES. DATE:	WED. DATE:
THURS. DATE:	FRI. DATE:	SAT. DATE:
		SUN. DATE:

MON. DATE:	TUES. DATE:	WED. DATE:

THURS. DATE:	FRI. DATE:	SAT. DATE:
		SUN. DATE:

MON. DATE:	TUES. DATE:	WED. DATE:

THURS. DATE:	FRI. DATE:	SAT. DATE:
		SUN. DATE:

MON. DATE:	TUES. DATE:	WED. DATE:

THURS. DATE:	FRI. DATE:	SAT. DATE:
		SUN. DATE:

MON. DATE:	TUES. DATE:	WED. DATE:

THURS. DATE:	FRI. DATE:	SAT. DATE:
		SUN. DATE:

MON. DATE:	TUES. DATE:	WED. DATE:
THURS. DATE:	FRI. DATE:	SAT. DATE:
		SUN. DATE:

MON. DATE:	TUES. DATE:	WED. DATE:
THURS. DATE:	FRI. DATE:	SAT. DATE:
		SUN. DATE:

MON. DATE:	**TUES.** DATE:	**WED.** DATE:

THURS. DATE:	**FRI.** DATE:	**SAT.** DATE:
		SUN. DATE:

MON. DATE:	**TUES.** DATE:	**WED.** DATE:

THURS. DATE:	**FRI.** DATE:	**SAT.** DATE:
		SUN. DATE:

MON. DATE:	**TUES.** DATE:	**WED.** DATE:
THURS. DATE:	**FRI.** DATE:	**SAT.** DATE:
		SUN. DATE:

MON. DATE:	**TUES.** DATE:	**WED.** DATE:
THURS. DATE:	**FRI.** DATE:	**SAT.** DATE:
		SUN. DATE:

MON. DATE:	**TUES.** DATE:	**WED.** DATE:
THURS. DATE:	**FRI.** DATE:	**SAT.** DATE:
		SUN. DATE:

MON. DATE:	**TUES.** DATE:	**WED.** DATE:
THURS. DATE:	**FRI.** DATE:	**SAT.** DATE:
		SUN. DATE:

MON. DATE:	**TUES.** DATE:	**WED.** DATE:
THURS. DATE:	**FRI.** DATE:	**SAT.** DATE:
		SUN. DATE:

MON. DATE:	**TUES.** DATE:	**WED.** DATE:
THURS. DATE:	**FRI.** DATE:	**SAT.** DATE:
		SUN. DATE:

NOTES

TOPICS/QUESTIONS TO CONSIDER ASKING YOUR DOCTOR

Curing or slowing your cancer is always the focus and priority of your medical team to ensure that you have a long and healthy life. When you first learn that you have cancer, that too is the center of your attention. As the days and weeks go by and you have more time to ponder what the future will bring, other questions may come to your mind. These questions are often about the quality of life that you can expect as you move to survivorship. This list is not exhaustive, each person is unique and will have goals and dreams that are specific to them. Feel free to add your thoughts to the list. The most important thing for you to know is that your medical team wants to know what is important to you. They want to help you conquer your cancer and to have a happy, fulfilling future.

1. **WHAT IS THE PLAN TO MANAGE ANY SYMPTOMS THAT I MAY EXPERIENCE?**

_____

_____

_____

_____

2. **IS MY CANCER HEREDITARY? DO I NEED TO WORRY ABOUT MY CHILDREN AND SIBLINGS?**

_____

_____

_____

_____

3. **DID YOU DO GENETIC OR MOLECULAR TESTING? DOES MY CANCER HAVE A MUTATION OR BIOMARKER? HOW DOES THAT HELP FIND THE BEST TREATMENT FOR ME?**

_____

_____

_____

_____

4. HOW WILL CANCER OR MY TREATMENT AFFECT MY JOB?

_____
_____
_____
_____

5. CAN I EXERCISE?

_____
_____
_____
_____

6. DO I NEED TO SEE A DENTIST? DO I NEED TO TELL THE
   DENTIST ABOUT MY CANCER AND TREATMENT?

_____
_____
_____
_____

7. ARE THERE SPECIAL FOODS THAT I SHOULD EAT WHILE HAVING
   TREATMENT? ARE THERE FOODS I SHOULD NOT EAT?

_____
_____
_____
_____

8. WILL I LOSE MY HAIR? WILL IT GROW BACK?

_____
_____
_____
_____

9. WILL I BE WEAK OR FATIGUED?

_____
_____
_____
_____

10. I HEAR PEOPLE TALKING ABOUT "CHEMO BRAIN".
    WHAT IS THAT AND WILL I GET IT?

_____
_____
_____
_____

11. WILL THE CANCER OR TREATMENT EFFECT MY
    SEXUAL HEALTH OR INTIMACY?

_____
_____
_____
_____

12. SHOULD I BE ON BIRTH CONTROL WHILE I AM ON TREATMENT?

_____
_____
_____
_____

13. WILL CANCER OR TREATMENT AFFECT MY FERTILITY?

_____
_____
_____
_____

14. SHOULD I STILL SEE MY PRIMARY CARE DOCTOR OR MY INTERNIST?

_____

_____

_____

_____

15. DO I STILL NEED OTHER CANCER SCREENING TESTS?

_____

_____

_____

_____

16. DOES MY FAMILY NEED TO TAKE ANY PRECAUTIONS WHEN I'M ON
    TREATMENT? IS IT OK TO BE AROUND MY CHILDREN/GRANDCHILDREN?

_____

_____

_____

_____

17.

_____

_____

_____

_____

18.

_____

_____

_____

_____

19.

20.

21.

22.

23.

NOTES

NOTES

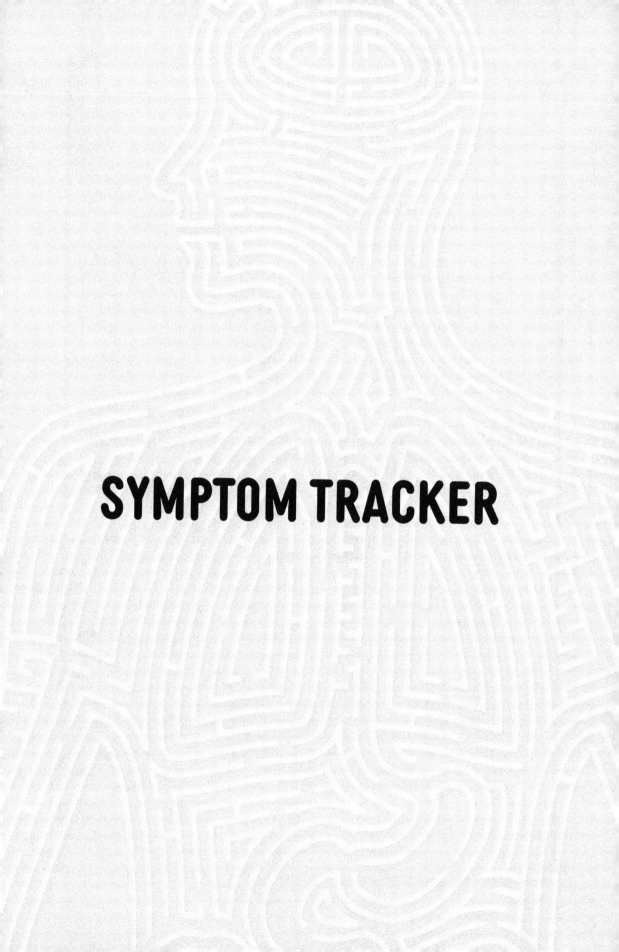

SYMPTOM TRACKER

How am I feeling? Different treatments may have different side effects and each person responds differently. Ask your nurse or doctor which symptoms you might expect. This is a list of some of the more common symptoms that you might experience after you begin treatment. Be sure to report any side effects that you have to your doctor:

DATE:	
	If you have a fever, call the oncologist's office immediately
	I have new or worsening pain
	I feel nausea or I am vomiting
	I feel dizzy or unusually weak
	I feel confused
	My appetite has changed
	I have difficulty sleeping
	I have sores in my mouth or on my lips
	I bruise easily and have an unusual number of bruises on my body
	My gums bleed when I brush my teeth
	I tire easily and am not able to do my normal daily activities
	My vision has changed
	My hearing has changed
	My speech has changed or I'm slurring my words
	I have difficulty finding the right words

	I have difficulty thinking
	I have headaches, more than usual
	I am forgetting things, my memory has changed
	I am angry, sad or feel down at times for no reason
	I have trouble walking
	I sometimes lose my balance or I have had a fall
	I have new weakness in my arms or legs
	My hands are shaky
	Redness, swelling or drainage from surgical wound
	I have hot flashes or night sweats or both

NOTES

NOTES

NOTES

NOTES

NOTES

NOTES

NOTES

NOTES

NOTES

CPSIA information can be obtained
at www.ICGtesting.com
Printed in the USA
BVHW020007260623
666349BV00008B/25